EXCLUSIVE BREAST FEEDING

HEALTHY NUTRITIONAL ACCEPTABLE WAYS OF CHILD FLOURISHING

BY

Dr. AMANDA FRAY

CONTENTS

CHAPTER ONE

INTRODUCTION

Exclusively breastfeeding infants from birth to 6 months of age ensures a safe, clean, healthy, accessible and uniquely tailored food source for nutritional needs wherever they live.

You can get latching the neonate within the first hour of life (known as early breastfeeding initiation) is critical for neonatal survival and long-term establishment of breastfeeding.

Postnatal delay in breastfeeding can be life threatening, and the longer a newborn waits, the higher the risk of death. Wherever they live, they can be assured of health, clean, healthy accessible food sources that are uniquely tailored to their nutritional needs.

Latching the neonate within the first hour of life (known as early breastfeeding initiation) is critical for neonatal survival and long-term establishment of breastfeeding.

Delayed breastfeeding after birth can have life-threatening consequences.

Also, the longer a newborn waits to be breastfed, the higher the risk of death and pneumonia than a newborn. Additionally, breastfeeding supports an infant's immune system and may protect against chronic diseases such as obesity and diabetes.

Have you ever wanted to exclusively breast feed your child?

Correct Failure to do so will result in loss of maternal health.

Exclusive breastfeeding has an air of natural intelligence and health that both mother and child enjoy.

Babies are exclusively breastfed from birth to six months of age.

During this period, it is recommended to exclusively breastfeed with no additional intake.

Exclusive breastfeeding has many benefits for your baby. A mother's joy when her baby is born is so heartwarming that she forgets her birth pains

With the above in mind, safely leading your baby to breastfeeding is crucial in providing your child with the nutrients they need to grow strong and healthy.

Breastfeeding is as old as mankind.

CHAPTER TWO

THE FIRST FOOD A BABY NEED TO EAT AFTER 6-MONTH

The first food a baby eats after conception is fortified breast milk given by the mother's so what can babies of 6 months give?

Babies can eat anything except honey, which they should not eat until they are one year old.

Healthy snacks like fruits purees can be added between meals.

As your baby eats more solids, he should continue to drink the same amount of milk.

Feeding a non-breastfed baby

if you are not breastfeeding your baby, your baby will need to eat more often.

She also has to rely on other foods, including dairy, to get all the nutrients her body needs.

Start feeding your baby solid foods as you would. Start with 2-3 spoonful of soft, pureed food four times a day.

This will give you the nutrients you need without breast milk.

• At 6-8 months, she needs 1/2 cup of soft food and healthy snacks 4 times a day.

• At 9-11 months, she needs 1/2 cup of food 4-5 times a day and she needs 2 healthy snacks.

9 months to 11 months Baby She can eat half a glass of food 3 to 4 times a day and healthy snacks.

She can now mince soft foods instead of grinding them

Babies may even start using their fingers to feed

themselves.

Continue breastfeeding when your baby is hungry.

• All meals should be baby-friendly and nutritious.

Cherish every bite.

• Food should be rich in energy and nutrients. In addition

to cereals and potatoes, make sure your baby eats

daily vegetables and fruits, legumes and seeds, energy-

rich oils and fats, and above all animal products (dairy

products, eggs, meat, fish and poultry).

Eating a variety of foods each day will

increase your chances of getting all the nutrients your

baby needs.

• If your baby refuses new food or vomits, do not force it. Please try again in a few days.

You can also mix it with other foods your baby likes and squeeze breast milk on top.

CHAPTER THREE

BREASTFEEDING BABIES: 1-2 YEARS

At this age, breast milk still provides important nutrients and protects against disease, but other foods become the primary source of nutrition and energy.

I'm here. Give other foods first, then breastfeed if still hungry.

Your child can eat anything, so give them all the food your family eats and cherish every bite.

Every meal should be packed with nutritious foods.

Aim for daily intake of animal products (milk, dairy products, eggs, meat, fish, poultry), legumes (example: chickpeas, lentils, peas) or nuts, orange or green vegetables, increase and fruit.

small amount of oil is added to the feed for energy.

Make sure your child's snacks are healthy.

Fresh fruit. Children can eat 3/4 to 1 cup of food and 1 to 2 snacks 3 to 4 times a day. If you don't breastfeed, you have to eat more often. By the time she's 1 year old when she starts walking, your child's meal plan should include 4-5 meals a day and 2 healthy snacks for her. Dairy products are a very important part of your child's diet.

Give her 1 or 2 cups of milk daily. Feeding Tips having their own bowl encourages kids to feed themselves. Start as soon as he wants.

Give him everything he needs and enough time. Slow and chaotic at first.

Help him get most of the food in his mouth (not on himself or on the floor!).Encourage him to finish and make sure he eats enough.

Give your child lots of love and encouragement about eating at mealtimes.

Sit in front of him and make eye contact. Interact with your kids, smile at them, talk to them, compliment their food

Make eating time a happy time!

Foods to Avoid

Avoid junk foods and soft drinks. Factory-made snacks such as chips, cookies, cakes, sodas, and candies are unhealthy, they are high in sugar, salt, fat, and chemicals, leaving your child's stomach space filled with nutritious foods.

Occupy what should I do if my child does not eat
solid foods?

Although breastfeeding is still healthy for your child, do
not breastfeed until after meals.

At this age, she should eat
solid foods first. Experiment with different food
combinations and textures.
If he still refuses, don't force him to eat or feed him junk
food instead.
Please take it easy. Give your child active attention
when he is eating, but ignore when he is not.
Remove the food, cover it, and give it back to her
a little later.

CHAPTER FOUR

THE MOST IMPORTANT THINGS PARENTS CAN DO TO SUPPORT BRAIN DEVELOPMENT

Supporting young child development, especially brain development the most important thing a parent can do to help is to know that young child, be able to read that child's signals, and get involved in what we "serve and give back". Serve and return is like a game. The reason "serve and return" describes exactly what is important in an interaction is that it is two-way. The baby smiles, coos, babbles, gestures, and the parent or other adult caring for the child returns responses that relate to what the baby did.

Baby makes noise they return the same sound.

Baby pointing at something you see it and you're

pointing to yourself. That's the key it goes both ways

in question.

A listening baby can start doing it. Parents can start.

What matters is how you react.

Serves and returns are not always successful on the

first try. But the more you practice, the easier it will

become. Start by turning your "serve and return" mindset

into something simple, familiar, and relaxing.

Play occurs when you are feeding your child, dressing

your child, or bathing your child.

These are all opportunities for playful interaction and

learning between adults and children.

To help parents understand that when they start

playing, they are actually building brain circuits, rather

than just regaining their smile and stopping there.

Why are baby words important?

Parents should immerse their babies more in Baby Talk,

which helps babies develop their own language skills.

Baby Talk works like a spotlight. Babies hear a lot of

sounds around them. But when you hear your baby's

words, you know it's time to listen and pay attention.

There are two reasons for this for her:

First, it makes it easier to hear the baby.

When babies are very young, they don't understand

the meaning of words. But they hear and learn from the

exaggerated pitches of baby talk.

Second, babies love to listen to babies. They like Baby

Talk's exaggerated melodic patterns and

positive sentiment.

This allows them to pay more attention to him compared

to the language we use towards adults.

Most people instinctively utter baby words when they see

a baby.

But it still doesn't come naturally to everyone. Parents

should start practicing baby talk early on to learn

what kind of baby talk to use.

The best time to practice baby language is when you are

going about your daily life with your baby.

For example, when eating, bathing, or playing with your

baby.

If you want to add a little more variety to your

statement, you can also describe a picture of a book or a

favorite toy your baby wants.

• Give your baby a chance to see you, hear you, move freely and touch you. You should be able to see the baby's limbs moving incoherently. Babies slowly learn to control their movements.

• Look into the baby's eyes and smile in response to the smile. You need to see your baby react positively to your facial expressions, movements and gestures.

• Speak "baby talk" in a baby-friendly tone. Both fathers and mothers, as well as other caregivers, need to communicate with their newborn. She can listen and will start memorizing and copying your words in no time.

• Change the tone of voice smoothly. Make it slow/fast, high/low or quiet/loud. You should observe how your baby reacts on his face and body and how he interacts with you.

• Soothe your child, pet him or give him a gentle

hug. You can see your

baby being comforted, happily held and cuddled.

• In contact with skin. Feeling, hearing and smelling your

presence should make your baby feel calm and safe

CHAPTER FIVE

PROACTIVE DISCIPLINE TO A CHILD

• "Parents don't want to yell at or hit their children. We do it because we are stressed and we don't see any other way around it.

• The evidence is clear. Yelling and punching have no effect and can cause harm over time. Repeated yelling and hitting can even affect a child for life.

The long-term "toxic stress" it creates can have a variety of adverse effects, including: Likely school dropout, depression, drug use, suicide, heart disease.

• "It's like saying, this is this drug. It doesn't work, it makes you sick, and if you know something is going wrong, that's good reason to look for a different approach."

• A positive discipline approach encourages interaction with your child, rather than punishing or disciplining. We focus on building healthy relationships and setting expectations about behavior.

• 1. Schedule a one-on-one session

• One-on-one sessions are important for building a good relationship. With your children. "It can be 20 minutes a day, or even five minutes. You can combine it with singing a song while washing the dishes together, or hanging out the laundry and chatting, what really matters is that you focus on her own child. Turn off her TV, turn off her cell phone, get on her level, and you and her

• 2. Praise the Positive

• As parents we often notice and name bad behavior in our children. Children can read this to get their attention and continue bad behavior instead of stopping it.

• Children grow when they are praised. It makes you feel loved and special. "When they do something good, even if it's only five minutes of playing with their siblings, pay attention and praise them,

• 3. Clear Setting Expectations

• "Telling people exactly what to do is much more effective than telling them what not to do, Kids may not understand what you're saying if you ask them not to mess up." Set high expectations and raise expectations. The likelihood that they will do what you ask.

4. Creative Distraction

• When children are struggling, distracting them with

more positive activities can be an effective strategy,

Distracting them from something else by changing

the subject, introducing them to a

game, taking them to another room, going for a

walk, etc. successfully redirects their

energy to positive behavior.

• Timing is also important. Distraction is also

about recognizing and taking action when something

goes wrong. Paying attention when

a child begins to be fidgety, irritable, or irritable, or when

two of her siblings are staring at the same toy, is a

potential situation where one of her helps relieve before

it becomes.

• 5. Use Calm Consequences

• Part of growth is learning that if you do something,

something can happen. Defining this for your child is a simple process of teaching them responsibility and encouraging better behavior.

• Give your child the opportunity to do the right thing by explaining the consequences of bad behavior. give. For example, if you want your child to stop scribbling on the wall, you can tell them to stop. This gives them a warning and an opportunity to change their behavior.

• If they don't stop, face the consequences calmly and without anger, "and trust yourself. It won't be easy!"

• Consistency is a key component of positive parenting. And that's how we make them real. "She can take a teenager off her phone for an hour, but it can be difficult to take her off for a week. Completely free. "They can imitate facial expressions, bump spoons into pots, and sing along.

•Interacting with Older Children

• Teenagers, like younger children, want to be praised

and seen as good people. Personal contact is still

important to them. "They love dancing together in the

room and talking about their favorite singers, They

don't always show it, but they do.

• When setting expectations, 'Let them help you

set the rules, Sit down with them and try to agree on what

they should and shouldn't do at home. It will also

help them determine what the

consequences of unacceptable behavior will be. By

participating in this process, they can know that you

understand that they are becoming independent beings of

their own.

www.ingramcontent.com/pod-product-compliance
Lightning Source LLC
Chambersburg PA
CBHW051727250726
48653CB00008B/3242